Dedication

"This book is dedicated to all those who aspire to attain good health and happiness through a life of wellness."

Table of Contents

Chapter 1: Introduction

I wrote this book in response to the growing issue of obesity, with the goal of creating a practical and enjoyable diet plan for rapid weight loss. In today's hectic life, loaded with stress and living under tremendous pressure, it is easy to gain weight but quite hard to lose it. The majority of people who gain weight over time keep trying different ways, but due to different reasons, their attempts to lose weight don't succeed much.

Understanding the common causes of weight gain is the first step towards addressing the issue. By identifying the reasons behind weight gain, you can develop an effective plan to tackle the problem and start your weight-loss journey. Those who are too busy often struggle to find time for physical activity, which is essential for burning excess calories. Unfortunately, their hectic schedules are frequently unavoidable, given the demands of work and personal responsibilities.

Eating unhealthy foods is one of the most common reasons for weight gain, which makes losing weight even harder when you have to go to work or study while managing other responsibilities like house chores, family obligations, social activities, and so on. Enjoying foods for pleasure and satisfaction can make them difficult to give up, as they often provide a sense of comfort and enjoyment. These include burgers, French fries, fried foods like fried chicken and brisket meat, processed foods like cookies, cakes, bakery items, salty snacks like chips and crackers, and all those sugary, oily, greasy, and overcooked foods.

Processed and unhealthy foods are highly addictive. Many people prioritize short-term satisfaction over long-term health consequences, indulging in foods that bring pleasure but harm their well-being. This behavior is irresponsible and neglects the importance of health consciousness. Being health-conscious means being mindful of the ingredients and nutritional value of the food we consume. By prioritizing nutrient-dense foods for their health benefits rather than solely for taste and flavor, we can cultivate a healthy relationship with food and develop sustainable eating habits. This approach allows us to maintain good health and weight without worry, as nutritious food becomes our primary focus.

The consequences of being overweight are not good for your health, and to ignore them makes things even worse with time. The common problems caused by excess weight are diabetes, high blood pressure, heart diseases, gout, arthritis, and high cholesterol. When the body is unable to cope with long-term neglect, it finally starts to show signs of wear and tear and develops health conditions that people have to live with for a long time.

Being overweight is an unpleasant experience, and no one wants to be obese. It's both physically and mentally bad to be overweight. People want to live happily, enjoy their lives, look nice and fit, and do whatever they like according to their needs and wishes. Thus, it's crucial to opt for a healthy diet that is sustainable and gentle on your body, protecting your health from harmful side effects. This approach ensures that you don't inadvertently create new health problems while trying to address existing ones. By making wise dietary choices, you can avoid exacerbating your current health issues and instead take a positive step towards overall well-being.

People have become so used to eating unhealthy foods on a daily basis on such a scale that imagining a life without these foods is unthinkable for them. Their reliance on these foods has become a significant obstacle to achieving weight loss. When they attempt to follow a diet by cutting out familiar foods, they often struggle to sustain it beyond a few days, succumbing to cravings for the unhealthy foods they're accustomed to. This vicious cycle of relapse repeatedly hinders their progress, making it challenging to adopt a healthier eating habit. That is why most people are unable to lose their weight or maintain it after losing it.

Achieving and maintaining physical fitness requires a disciplined lifestyle that incorporates healthy habits, enabling you to enjoy overall wellness and a strong physical condition. Whenever people make unhealthy choices, they pay dearly for them. There are no excuses for ignoring one's health. Your health is totally in your hands, so you can either live a healthy life by taking care of it or ignore it; it is all up to you. There is no one else to blame for self-created problems.

The psychology behind weight gain and unsuccessful attempts to lose weight depends on factors like the complexities of modern lifestyles and the consumer society in which we live. The power of advertising is immense. Massive advertising of unhealthy foods is prevalent everywhere, including billboards, the internet, and print and electronic media like TV, making it evident that people are unable to resist the temptation to eat them.

Not everyone has the willpower to resist unhealthy foods immediately. Adopting a disciplined lifestyle that includes healthy eating habits can be challenging. Moreover, some individuals use unhealthy foods as a coping mechanism for emotional struggles like stress, unhappiness, depression, relationship issues, or loneliness. Therefore, understanding the underlying reasons behind their dependence on unhealthy foods is crucial to addressing the root cause of their habits.

Once you identify the underlying reasons driving your consumption of unhealthy foods, you can begin addressing the root causes and develop strategies to find satisfaction and pleasure in healthier ways. Working on a bigger problem requires a lot of work and a complete plan to follow. However, achieving such transformations requires unwavering commitment and dedication to your goals. While obstacles are inevitable, working through them is crucial to overcoming them. With determination and hard work, you can overcome any obstacle and achieve a fulfilling life of purpose and success.

Weight loss can have a profoundly transformative impact on one's life, leading to a radical transformation that affects almost every aspect. The benefits of weight loss are numerous and significant, ranging from improved physical health to enhanced mental well-being and a boost in overall quality of life. People who lose weight look happier, healthier, satisfied, and full of energy. They live their lives to the fullest by reaping the rewards of their successful weight-loss achievements. Those who achieve weight loss don't want to gain weight again.

The timing and scheduling of our meals have a profound impact on our body's internal clock and overall health. Similarly, it affects our body's weight regulation. So adjusting our meal times to the body's internal system in the right way benefits our health and keeps us in good shape. Eating properly, healthy, and on time is the key to good health and fitness. Staying in shape demands taking care of every aspect that is important for our health. When we take care of our health, we are the ones who benefit, and when we ignore it, we pay the price.

There is not an easy solution for a long-term problem. Either you'll succeed in achieving and sustaining weight loss, or you'll face an ongoing struggle to reach your weight goals. It is more of a choice and decision that people have to make, whether they want to make serious changes in their lives by working on them or leave things as they are. What's the point of continuing to struggle with weight loss using ineffective methods when you could be taking a proven approach to achieve sustainable success? Once you understand this point, you are going to eventually achieve your weight-loss goal.

Losing weight slowly or rapidly all depends on your decision. If you want to lose weight rapidly, you can do so, just like others who do it. There is nothing that can stop you once you make up your mind. So the first thing to do is to make a decision. Losing weight starts the day you follow a diet with your heart and mind. You must be fully committed and determined. Clear your mind of all the doubt that you can't lose weight. Your past struggles with weight loss are fueling your current doubts. But the past is the past, and what really matters is your present and future.

If past weight loss attempts failed due to inconsistency and impatience, it's essential to overcome these obstacles to achieve successful and rapid weight loss this time around. Stop thinking about short cuts or easy ways; such thinking deprives people of achieving success. Combine your efforts with time, dedication, motivation, and consistency, and nothing can stop you from losing your weight rapidly. Healthy food choices do the heavy lifting, while regular exercise and physical activity fill in the gaps on the path to a healthier lifestyle.

People not only want to reduce their extra weight, but what they really want is to do so as soon as possible in an easy way. It's all about choosing the best possible option that is available to them— the one they can't refuse. This explains why there is a high demand for weight loss methods that promise quick and rapid results, as people seek fast solutions to achieve their weight goals. But the important thing not to forget is to choose the healthiest possible options that enable rapid weight loss, so that it is a win-win situation.

The key to successful weight loss is to approach it in a sustainable way that promotes long-term maintenance. Rather than trying fad diets that only lead to temporary weight reduction, followed by regaining the weight, it's essential to adopt a realistic and sustainable approach. This means learning to incorporate healthy foods and lifestyle habits into your daily routine, making it possible to maintain weight loss permanently. By focusing on sustainable changes, individuals can break the cycle of yo-yo dieting and achieve a healthier weight for the long haul.

It is frustrating to keep trying different diets and be unable to reduce weight to the desired level. The more you try different diets without completing them, the more you get used to trying diets on a short-term basis. It's like being stuck in a vicious cycle of weight loss and gain by repeating the same mistake, making it difficult to achieve lasting success. It's a hopeless situation for many people who are struggling to lose weight. The more their attempts to lose weight are fruitless, the more they start to believe that their goal of losing weight is unattainable, and eventually they give up and pay more attention to their daily existence and other matters of life.

Both malnutrition and overnutrition are harmful for health. The best way is to find balance and consume only what your body needs. Whenever you don't give your body what it needs, it results in health problems. Eating too little can lead to malnutrition, causing fatigue, weakness, and various health problems due to inadequate nutrition. Conversely, overindulging in unhealthy foods can result in obesity, triggering a range of health issues and mental wellbeing concerns, ultimately significantly impacting quality of life.

Many people are unaware of the harmful effects of irregular eating habits, such as skipping meals, eating at random times, and ignoring hunger cues. These habits can lead to a weak digestive system and various health issues. However, establishing a consistent eating schedule can help regulate digestion and promote overall well being. Our stomach isn't a machine that can run 24/7; it needs care and attention to function optimally. By prioritizing digestive health, you can ensure your body receives the necessary nutrients to stay healthy and strong.

Those who disregard their health by neglecting its fundamental needs ultimately make their lives more difficult. The body can only tolerate so much neglect and mistreatment before it begins to break down, leading to deteriorating health. It's essential to treat your body with kindness and respect, as neglecting your health only leads to harmful consequences. Why not behave responsibly and take care of your health? Well, these are the things people need to think about seriously.

The manufacturers of unhealthy foods don't care about the impact of the foods they are selling on the health of people because they are only interested in making profits. Similarly, restaurants, fast food chains, and cafes often prioritize taste and pleasure over nutritional value, glossing over the health implications of their offerings. These businesses sell unhealthy food at high prices to make a profit. People pay a high price for their mistakes when they choose to eat tasty but unhealthy food.

Some people mistakenly believe that consuming light meals is ineffective and leads to rapid hunger. However, this assumption is far from the truth. Another misconception is that light meals and natural foods don't really provide what the body needs in terms of vitamins, proteins, and nourishment. Both of these beliefs are wrong. Light meals and healthy foods are filling, provide you with enough energy and nourishment, and keep you healthy and strong on a long-term basis.

People have gotten used to the fast lifestyle because everyone wants a quick solution to their problem and wants to get things done as soon as possible. This mindset is also influencing people's food choices and dietary habits. People just want to grab something to eat quickly, ignoring the health implications, quality, and health effects of foods. This is causing obesity. The older the habits are, the harder it is to get rid of them.

Lifestyle changes need a lot of work and determination. People either lack motivation to bring about changes or leave things as they are because of their own laziness or ignorance. The combination of these factors makes life harder. Unfortunately, many people struggle to understand that meaningful change, including weight loss, requires a transformation in lifestyle and eating habits. Until they make these changes, they'll face obstacles to achieving their goals and improving their lives.

Everyone who is overweight wants to get in shape, but many are unwilling to do the work that requires that achievement. Many individuals struggle with weight issues for an extended period of time, making it a persistent problem. Unfortunately, most people wait too long to take action, allowing the issue to persist and become a long-term struggle. Instead of waiting when things get out of control, the right way to do things is to start doing it before it gets too late.

Health should be a top priority for everyone, as it is a vital aspect of our lives that cannot be ignored or neglected. Poor health disrupts life's balance and has a ripple effect, making things worse. As we all know, good health is essential for a happy, productive, and fulfilling life, and ignoring our health can have serious consequences. So instead of postponing further weight loss plans, start immediately to take the steps that will help you lose your weight quickly before some health issues can make your life difficult.

For sustainable weight loss, a carefully designed diet prioritizes both rapid progress and long-term wellbeing, enabling swift and healthy weight reduction for all. This approach focuses on whole, natural foods and a healthy lifestyle, recognizing that the best way to lose weight is through balanced eating and regular physical activity. By incorporating healthy habits into their daily routine, individuals can efficiently and safely achieve weight loss goals, leveraging the combined benefits of nutritious food and regular exercise to accelerate progress.

Rapid weight loss works when you make it work by first understanding it well. By adopting a balanced diet and a healthy lifestyle, weight loss becomes a sustainable and rapid achievement, leading to long-term results that benefit overall health and wellbeing. By embracing wholesome foods and habits, you'll experience long-term benefits and find it easier to maintain a healthy weight. As you cultivate a taste for nutritious foods and a healthy lifestyle, you'll find it becomes second nature, making it simpler to sustain your weight loss journey in the long run. It's not an easy-come, easy-go thing because when you achieve something with some effort, it has long-lasting benefits that truly help you.

It's important to recognize that meaningful achievements require effort and dedication. Long-term benefits, such as successful weight loss, are rarely the result of quick fixes or miracles. Instead, they require commitment to healthy habits and lifestyle changes. If you're waiting for a magic solution to achieve weight loss without making any changes, you'll likely be disappointed. Sustainable weight loss demands a willingness to adapt your eating habits and lifestyle choices. Doing things the wrong way doesn't produce any positive results. Many individuals face a frustrating cycle of weight loss and regain known as 'yo-yo dieting.' This occurs when they fail to maintain healthy eating habits and lifestyle changes after initial weight loss, leading to a return to unhealthy patterns and regaining weight. Breaking this cycle requires a long-term commitment to sustainable lifestyle choices, rather than temporary fixes.

Your motivation, inner strength, and self-control are your biggest assets that help you live a disciplined life. People who possess certain qualities are more likely to lead successful lives. Among these qualities, one of the most essential is belief in oneself. When it comes to weight loss, believing in your ability to achieve your goals is the first and most crucial step. With self-belief, you'll be more motivated to make healthy lifestyle changes and stay committed to your weight-loss journey.

Before starting this diet, please consult your doctor to ensure it's suitable for your individual health needs and circumstances. If you have food allergies, carefully review the diet's food options to avoid any potential allergens. The good news is that this diet doesn't require fasting or extreme exercise, making it accessible to a wide range of ages and health conditions. By consulting your doctor and taking the necessary precautions, you can safely and confidently embark on this diet and reap its benefits. The diet is based on eating healthy, light, and natural foods to achieve weight loss really fast without going through any hardships.

Chapter 2: Understanding This Diet

This diet is based on the principle that whatever you eat should be natural, lighter, and easy to digest, and you should make your own portion size according to your appetite. This is absolutely not a starvation diet that requires fasting, small food portions, or restricting the choice of foods to a minimum amount. Due to these qualities, this diet makes it easier to follow by eating foods from the healthy range while still being able to reduce weight quickly and safely.

The diet's approach is to provide your body with only the necessary calories, minimizing surplus energy, by combining healthy foods with tailored physical activity aligned to your individual capacity to achieve rapid weight loss. The diet allows you to eat freely from the permitted list of foods to provide sufficient nourishment, vitamins, proteins, and energy to live a normal and healthy life.

This diet offers a comfortable and sustainable solution for those who struggle with extreme fasting or unrealistic exercise demands. By swapping unhealthy foods for nutrient-dense options and embracing a balanced lifestyle, you'll unlock the power to achieve your weight-loss goals and transform your overall health. Unlike restrictive approaches, this diet fosters lasting change, helping you progress towards a healthier outcome.

While munching throughout the day may work for some, it's important to remember that our stomachs aren't machines that can run non-stop. Constantly eating can exhaust our digestive system, making it less efficient and stealing time away from productivity. Instead, let's optimize our eating habits to balance nutrition, digestive health, and time management—a better way to achieve our goals without wearing out our bodies.

It's not just about what you eat; it also counts when you eat. So timing plays an important role, along with choosing the right types of foods that are good for your health. It's all about the winning combination, just like in sports. A team with a good combination scores the win. Just like that, this is the winning formula created to help you lose weight with this diet.

Let the day be for eating and physical activity, and reserve the evening to morning hours for rest and fasting, avoiding food intake when your body is at rest. This approach allows you to fuel your body during active hours and optimize digestion, growth, and repair during rest. Let's say you stop eating around 6 p.m. until the morning, when you usually eat your breakfast. You'll see the pounds melt away as this approach helps you achieve your weight-loss goals!

Making things easy or difficult is all up to you. Consuming unhealthy foods and adopting a sedentary lifestyle can lead to weight gain. If you start eating foods high in sugar, grease, fat, spice, salt, and processed ingredients and abandon healthy habits, you'll notice a significant weight gain in just a few weeks. You will feel tired, lazy, and stressed. But just when you do the opposite—eat healthy and be physically active—and you see how you get in great shape, your level of energy and happiness will always be high. You will feel totally different than before.

When the facts are clear, it's time to take control of your health! With the truth about healthy and unhealthy habits in plain sight, there's no reason to delay making a positive change. Start eating healthy and living healthy today; your body and mind will be grateful to you. Just overcome your shortcomings and motivate yourself to start changing your life without any further delay.

When we let our weaknesses take hold of our lives, we make them difficult. Eating unhealthy foods is a human weakness and a mistake that surely costs you a lot. You can't keep indulging in unhealthy foods and expect to lose weight—it's time to align your eating habits with your goals! Doing things the wrong way doesn't produce positive results; it's as simple as that. When you understand this, you are going to start making big changes in your life with long-term positive implications for your life.

When you eat light meals and soups, you see how quickly they start to show their positive results. Let light meals work for you, and soon you will see the results coming in. A combination of light meals made from natural and healthy foods, accompanied by salads, soups, fruits, and plenty of water and juice, can help you lose weight quickly and easily. It's like making a setup and letting it do its work for you.

The light meals fill you and give you energy and proteins without any surplus of calories, thus making the process of reducing weight a reality. It's like pin-pointing a problem. You remove bad foods and replace them with healthy ones. That's all you have to do, and the results will be so heartwarming for you that you will not be able to hide your happiness and excitement.

A healthy eating regime is the key to weight loss. By sticking to a regular schedule for breakfast, lunch, and dinner, your body's internal clock adjusts, and your digestive system functions at its optimal level, leading to improved overall health and well-being. A fixed interval between meal times helps our digestive system function properly. A longer overnight break between your early dinner and the morning breakfast does the work by giving your body the rest it needs after the whole day of work.

Eating a light meal early in the evening can help you maintain a healthy weight by reducing your overall calorie intake. Additionally, avoiding heavy meals close to bedtime can also prevent heartburn and acidity, promoting a more comfortable and restful night's sleep. The more your body is at peace at night, the better your sleep quality will be, and your next day will be full of productivity.

The key to success in this diet lies in calorie restriction, as excessive calorie intake is the main reason behind weight gain. By limiting calories, you create a deficit that sparks rapid weight loss. No extra calories means no more weight gain. To lose weight, it's essential to strike a balance between the calories you consume and the calories your body burns. When you maintain a reasonable calorie deficit, your body begins to tap into stored fat for energy, leading to rapid weight loss. The key is to fuel your body with a balanced diet that provides the necessary nutrients to support this process. By eating healthy foods and burning the right amount of calories, you'll be on track to achieve your weight-loss goals.

This diet recognizes a common hurdle in weight loss: the struggle to maintain a diet over time. For those who are overweight, this challenge often leads to a persistent weight problem. Despite their best intentions, individuals may find it difficult to adhere to a diet for an extended period, making it hard to achieve sustainable weight loss. By acknowledging this common obstacle, this diet seeks to offer a more effective and sustainable weight-loss solution.

Following a diet is not easy without strong motivation, dedication, patience, and continuity. Not all diets are suitable for everyone, and switching between diets without commitment doesn't lead to different results. Thus, this diet is carefully designed to be easy to follow and stick to, ensuring successful weight loss from start to finish. All you have to do is eat only from the permitted list of foods, eat light meals, drink plenty of liquids, and take part in some physical activities to keep yourself active and make this diet produce rapid results for you.

This diet has a positive impact on mental well-being, as it is comfortable and sustainable, promoting happiness and overall wellness. In fact, it does the opposite. By following this diet, you feel happy and upbeat that you are eating healthy foods without fasting or other strict measures that are not easy for everyone to follow. The light meals, together with fresh fruits, salads, juices, and other natural foods, make this diet enjoyable with a happy-go effect.

It's a low-calorie diet that does its work efficiently. Low-calorie foods don't let the body build up extra calories that it does not need, thus leaving less work for the body to do to shed those surplus calories, thus making it difficult to build up fat in the body. The more you ease your body into calorie adjustments, the better and more sustainable your results will be. That's the core principle of this diet.

Natural foods are not only easy to digest but also provide nourishment, unlike processed foods that are high in calories and take longer to digest. People who eat natural foods look fresh and energetic. Their skin looks good, and they are overall healthy and happy.

So when you eat lighter meals made of natural produce and ingredients, it helps you in many ways to stay fit, healthy, and in good shape. Eating nutritious foods has numerous benefits, leading to a more comfortable and convenient life, both physically and mentally.

Choosing this diet is crucial because it supports digestive health, which has far-reaching benefits for the body and mind. By incorporating easily digestible foods into your diet, you'll support immune function, increase energy levels, and enjoy a profound enhancement of mental well-being. This diet's focus on easy digestion optimizes overall health and mental well-being.

This diet was created to accelerate weight loss. Once you start seeing results, it will give you a lot of encouragement. The encouragement that comes with tracking your progress will help you stay committed to your goals. As you begin to shed pounds, the diet's natural, fresh, light, and flavorful foods will help you gain momentum, achieving your desired weight in a short time.

Chapter 3: Rules for the Diet

Every diet has some rules, and so does this one. In this diet, some foods are left out on purpose because the goal is to see quick results. The reasons why these foods are excluded are explained in detail:

Wheat

Refined Sugar and Artificial Sweeteners

Excessive Use of Sodium

Butter

Processed Foods

Overcooked Foods

Red Meat

Alcohol

Oily, Greasy, and Fried Foods

Potatoes

Wheat:

Wheat is a ubiquitous ingredient, found in a wide range of foods, including bread, cookies, fast food, snacks, and sweets, making it a common component of many diets. It is a staple food around the world. Bread is a staple food in many cultures, with millions of tons of wheat harvested annually to meet global demand. While moderate consumption of healthier bread options is unlikely to lead to weight gain, excessive intake of flour-based products throughout the day can lead to weight gain and potentially hinder weight loss efforts. Bread and wheat products are not only commonly eaten but are also part of many meals, from breakfast to dinner. It's important to keep a check on the amount of food you eat.

Eating refined wheat products like bakery items, snacks, or desserts can lead to weight gain. Bread, a common food eaten daily by many people, can lead to weight gain if consumed daily.

Wheat has a high glycemic index, which causes a rapid spike in blood sugar. Not only does wheat disturb insulin levels, but it also has some addictive properties. Because of this, people easily develop the habit of consuming various wheat-based products regularly. That makes weight gain unavoidable.

There are some weight-loss diets where wheat is totally forbidden. That is called a gluten-free diet. There are people who have gluten allergies, but many people try this diet to reduce weight, which does help people reduce their weight. Hence, wheat is excluded from this diet to aid in rapid weight loss. Rice and other grains are great substitutes for wheat, like buckwheat, corn flour, and barley. Fortunately, wheat can be easily substituted with other nutritious grains that support weight loss goals, such as barley, quinoa, and brown rice.

Refined Sugar and Artificial Sweeteners:

Losing weight can be particularly challenging when trying to avoid foods and beverages containing refined sugar and artificial sweeteners. These ingredients are ubiquitous in processed foods, fizzy drinks, energy drinks, and other products, making them difficult to evade. Their widespread availability and aggressive marketing make it hard to resist their temptation, making weight loss even more daunting.

The common sources that are known for refined sugar are table sugar, high-fructose corn syrup, and fruit-flavored beverages. Artificial sweeteners, synthetic substitutes for refined sugar, are ubiquitous in a broad range of products, including sugar-free beverages, diet sodas, desserts, and low-calorie foods. These products are often marketed as healthier alternatives, despite ongoing debates about the potential health impacts of artificial sweeteners.

People often eat high-sugar foods without realizing it, leading to weight gain and health problems. Foods high in sugar and fat spike insulin in our body, which makes it difficult for our body to cope with the impact of excessive sugar, resulting in the formation of fat in our bodies and increasing the risk of getting diabetes. So this is what contributes to weight gain. Insulin does play a role in how our bodies handle food; it's just one of those factors when it comes to managing weight. Eating a balanced diet and staying active do their part of the work very efficiently.

Consuming refined sugar is a caloric and potentially weight-gain-inducing habit. Often overlooked is the fact that natural foods, like fruits, inherently contain sugars and can satisfy our taste and nutritional needs without the harmful effects of artificially processed sweeteners. Unlike refined sugar, which undergoes a chemical process that makes it unhealthy, fruits are naturally sweet and safe to consume, making them a great alternative choice.

Excessive Use of Sodium:

Though sodium is an essential part of our food, excessive use of salt makes it difficult to lose weight. Just like any other food, excessive use of salt has negative consequences for health. Overconsumption of salt makes the liquids stay in our body for a longer period of time and can cause kidney stones to form. Overconsumption of salt is a major reason for high blood pressure and heart disease. Many individuals regularly consume foods high in sodium, such as fast foods, potato chips, and crackers, often unaware of the potential health risks associated with excessive sodium intake, including blood pressure issues and cardiovascular disease.

Sodium is naturally present in vegetables and other whole foods, making a moderate amount of salt sufficient for health needs. This emphasizes the importance of balanced consumption, as excessive salt intake can lead to health issues like high blood pressure and cardiovascular disease. When there is table salt on the dining table at home or at restaurants, people put it on the food just to increase the flavor, thus making their food unhealthy.

Too much salt is commonly added in the food industry, especially in restaurants, fast food chains, and even airline meals, mainly to make the food taste better. This widespread practice contributes to the overconsumption of sodium, posing health risks to consumers. High blood pressure is a common problem, and that is due to the widespread use of salt in foods, even though everyone knows the risks of its excessive use. In a weight-loss diet, only a small amount of salt is allowed to help with the process. Consuming too much salt can cause bloating, making it hard to burn stomach fat and achieve a flatter stomach. This highlights the importance of salt intake moderation to support effective weight loss. Eating salty food during the evening hours is unhealthy and bad for the digestive system.

Butter:

Though butter has a lot of health qualities and is very tasty, it has a lot of fat in it. Butter is high in saturated fats, calories, and cholesterol. Excessive consumption can contribute to weight gain, obesity, and an increased risk of heart disease. So the use of butter is definitely not advised when you want to lose weight quickly. The fat ratio in butter is quite high, and when you are already overweight, there is no need to use butter. Instead of butter, use low-fat dairy products like cheddar cheese, milk, and yogurt.

Why use butter when there are better alternatives available when you are trying to lose weight? There are healthy vegetable oils

available and some great alternatives, like olive and avocado oil,
to do the job. Butter can be used in moderation when you want to
maintain your ideal weight; therefore, butter definitely should be
avoided when you want to lose weight rapidly.

Processed Foods:

Processed foods are a common convenience, but they come at a
cost. Regular consumption of these altered foods is a significant
contributor to weight gain. Whole foods are rich in nutrients and
health benefits, but processing and altering them can remove
these benefits, leaving behind a less healthy version. To achieve
weight loss and support overall health, it's essential to prioritize
natural foods over processed options, recognizing the significant
difference between these two categories. These foods are heavy
on the stomach and weaken the digestive system for a longer
period of time. Those who eat processed foods regularly easily
gain weight and lack energy and stamina.

When you go to a grocery store, you're surrounded by lots of
processed foods like cookies, candies, chocolates, baked goods,

cakes, pastries, and many other similar items. So imagine how difficult it must be for people to avoid buying these unhealthy foods while they are there. The attractive displays of these foods on shelves and counters are really tempting, making them difficult to resist.

When natural foods are processed into final products, they often include unhealthy ingredients like preservatives, artificial colors, flavor enhancers, and sweeteners. This manufacturing process, aimed at extending shelf life and enhancing flavor, unfortunately turns healthy foods into unhealthy ones, contributing to obesity and various health issues.

Some examples of processed foods are packaged snacks, canned foods, frozen meals, processed meats, and a wide range of different foods. Processed foods are bad for the liver and cause toxicity in the body. The obvious signs of an unhealthy liver and toxicity in the body are bad skin, acne, dandruff, tiredness, constipation, and stress. Despite knowing the potential health risks, people still find themselves drawn to these foods, often indulging in them anyway.

Processed foods are nothing else but full of added sugars, saturated fats, and refined carbs. Regularly consuming these foods means inviting health conditions like obesity, diabetes, heart disease, and certain cancers. So, just because these foods are easy to prepare and ready to eat makes them an attractive choice. They can often be cheaper than whole foods. They are addictive because their high taste makes them irresistible. So the only way to keep away from these foods is to look at the facts—not the convenience and taste, but what is healthy to eat.

Overcooked Foods:

In addition to the detrimental effects of oily and greasy foods, overcooked foods also present health concerns. Overcooking not only diminishes the nutritional content of foods but can also produce harmful compounds. High cooking temperatures can lead to the formation of carcinogens and advanced glycation end products (AGEs), which are associated with increased cancer risk and accelerated aging, respectively.

Furthermore, overcooked foods may lose their natural flavors and textures, resulting in less enjoyable eating experiences. Regular consumption of overcooked foods has been linked to digestive issues and nutrient deficiencies. Therefore, it is advisable to avoid overcooking foods and opt for healthier cooking methods such as steaming, baking, or grilling to preserve their nutritional value and minimize health risks.

Read Meat:

Red meat is tasty, highly nutritious, has a lot of proteins, and produces a lot of calories in the body. There are a wide variety of dishes prepared with beef, mutton, and lamb meat. Beef is widely used in fast food, like burgers. Grilled or BBQ meat, steaks, or jerky—there are a wide variety of tasty dishes all made of red meat. Red meat is a rich source of protein, minerals like zinc and iron, and vitamins B6 and B12. But on the other hand, due to being high in saturated fats, cholesterol, and calories, you can easily gain weight.

Although there are healthy options like sirloin, tenderloin, or round, which are low in fat and calories, you should only use them moderately to maintain your weight and not during the time you are following this diet. The real bad options when it comes to red meat are sausages, bacon, and deli meats, which are high in added sugars, salt, and unhealthy fats. Eating red meat spikes insulin levels and increases cholesterol in the body. Excessive use of red meat causes diabetes, gout, and arthritis.

There is a great alternative available in this diet to red meat, which is poultry, fish, and low-fat dairy products. The ideal alternative to red meat in this diet is chicken or turkey breast or fish like salmon, carp, tuna, and trout. Eggs are healthy and wonderful to provide your body with energy and nutrition; they should be part of your daily breakfast.

Alcohol:

Alcohol and weight loss are incompatible partners. Therefore, abstaining from alcohol is essential for effective weight loss. Consumption of alcohol can lead to addiction, posing risks to both health and personal well-being. With various types such as beer, wine, whisky, gin, and brandy, alcohol is prevalent in many cultures.

Alcohol is calorie-dense and promotes weight gain by stimulating appetite, often resulting in overeating. Those with prolonged alcohol issues struggle to manage their weight effectively. Beer consumption, especially during meals, contributes to the notorious "beer belly" phenomenon, expanding the waistline.

Additionally, alcohol hampers metabolism, hindering calorie burning. Long-term alcohol abuse can inflict liver damage, elevate cancer and heart disease risks, and trigger nutritional deficiencies and mental health issues. Given these detrimental effects, refraining from alcohol is a prudent choice for both physical and mental well-being.

Oily, Greasy, and Fried Foods:

There is a lot of talk about the link between fast food and obesity. No one can deny the fact that greasy and fast foods are responsible for weight gain. When hunger strikes, it's tempting to opt for quickly available fast food, which may provide instant gratification but can have long-term detrimental effects on your health.

These foods are usually cooked using unhealthy methods, which greatly lowers their nutritional value and makes them even more harmful to our health. They are too oily, which is bad for the digestive system. They give pleasure, but they also contribute to weight gain, increase toxicity in the body, increase stress, and reduce the body's natural capabilities. Popular fast foods such as pizzas, fried chicken, burgers, wraps, and French fries are loaded with calories and unhealthy fats. While they're tempting to your taste buds, they ultimately result in weight gain and raised cholesterol levels. The frying process further exacerbates their unhealthiness, providing no nutritional value whatsoever.

Using an excessive amount of oil in cooking makes foods unhealthy, and the digestive system finds them hard to digest. Eating fried and oily foods frequently can lead to oily skin and toxins in the body. Also, regularly consuming greasy, overcooked, and heavily seasoned foods, which are high in spices and sodium, can cause fatty liver disease.

Once you develop a taste for unhealthy foods, it's easy to overlook their harmful effects until you start experiencing negative health consequences. So, why wait until health problems force you to make a change? Take control of your diet and make healthier choices before it's too late. Why not do it before you start to have health problems?

Therefore, it's essential to completely avoid consuming overcooked, fried foods, and all types of fast food, which are notorious for providing excessive calories that are hard to burn, leading to weight gain and increased body fat. The global rise of fast food consumption has become a significant contributor to the alarming rate of obesity worldwide. Therefore, one should know the consequences of consuming these foods.

Potatoes:

Potatoes are likely the most commonly consumed vegetable globally. Potatoes are a staple food in many countries; they are quite popular in Europe and North America. Potatoes are a nutritional and versatile food cooked in many different ways and are a favorite food for many people. Millions of tons of potatoes are harvested every year around the world. Potatoes can be beneficial for health but can also be detrimental, depending on the preparation methods and consumption.

Potatoes are a rich source of fiber, potassium, vitamin C, and antioxidants. They are low in fat and calories. Potatoes themselves are healthy, but what affects their health properties is the preparation method. Cooking them in an unhealthy way can add extra calories, sodium, and fat. Unfortunately, potatoes are often cooked in an unhealthy way, especially when they're fried in oil. This can make them lose their nutritional value. Some of the most popular varieties of cooked potatoes are French fries, roast, mashed, and potato chips. Frying potatoes to create French fries and potato chips enhances their flavor but can negatively impact health due to the addition of excess fat and salt.

Potatoes have lots of carbohydrates, mainly starch, which can make blood sugar go up quickly. That's why they're not part of this diet. The best way to cook potatoes to keep them healthy is by boiling them and mixing them with other veggies.

The minimum or no use of oil during cooking makes potatoes a healthier option. Only cooking them in a healthy manner makes potatoes a healthy food. Eating potatoes in moderation and cooking them in a healthy way can help you maintain a healthy weight.

Chapter 4: Foods Permitted for Diet

This diet excludes foods that hinder weight loss and includes only those that accelerate the weight-loss process. This makes this diet ideal for those who want rapid weight loss without fasting or doing rigorous exercises. The main feature that makes it a suitable diet for everyone is that you can eat as much as you want from the permitted list of foods and don't worry about health risks, as this diet is based on health principles. Here is the list of foods that are permitted to be included in this diet:

Vegetables

Fruits

Legumes

Beans

Low-Fat Dairy Products

Eggs

Lean Meat

Dry Fruits

Seeds

Nuts

Grains

Vegetables:

Vegetables top this list due to their exceptional health benefits and significant role in facilitating weight loss. Rich with vitamins, minerals, fiber, and proteins, they provide the essential nutrition our body needs. One of the remarkable aspects of vegetables is their ability to provide ample energy for the body's needs despite being low in calories. Vegetables have a high liquid ratio, which makes them easy to cook and easy to digest.

Diets centered around vegetables are ideal for weight loss and weight maintenance, offering a safe option for promoting overall health. With a wide variety of vegetables accessible year-round, they provide a convenient and nutritious choice for everyday meals. Whether fresh or frozen, they are quick to prepare at home or are a healthy option when you eat them at restaurants. Fresh vegetables are great for making salads. Various types of salads can be prepared at home or enjoyed at restaurants.

Cultivating your own vegetables in your garden not only ensures a fresh and healthy supply but also serves as an engaging hobby and promotes physical activity. Vegetables grow quickly and are ideal for making homemade pickles. They offer versatility in cooking methods, including baking, roasting, grilling, boiling, or incorporating them into stews. Their aroma and taste are appetizing. Considering all these qualities and health properties, vegetables are indeed a great choice for rapid weight loss.

Fruits:

When it comes to fresh food, fruits are an all-time favorite for everyone. Everyone likes the taste and smell of fresh fruits. Just like vegetables, they are available all year. Whether it is summer or winter, there is a wide variety of fruits that come in different seasons all year round. Modern logistics and international trade have made the import and export of fruits easy. Fruits sourced from distant locations are readily available at local grocery stores or markets, offering convenience to consumers.

Citrus fruits are great for weight loss; they burn fat effectively and cleanse your body from toxic substances. Fresh citrus fruits like oranges, mandarins, grapefruit, lemons, and limes are great to eat, and you can make fresh juices from them.

Fresh fruit juices, milk shakes, fruit salads, or eaten in their original form make them a favorite food for all. What makes each fruit distinct from the others is that each one has a different taste, color, and size. Every person has their own favorite fruit. Some people like bananas, some like apples, so there is a wide variety available to choose from.

They are rich in fiber, vitamins, and minerals, which makes them an ideal choice for weight loss. They are low in calories and have natural sweetness, which is sufficient to fulfill the needs of the body. They are easily digestible and have great health properties. They are light and good for the digestive system. They clean the stomach, detoxify the body, increase stamina, make you healthier, and lift up your mood.

Eating fruits makes it easy to lose and maintain weight. Eating a few fruits every day keeps you healthy, fresh, energetic, and happy. Freshly consumed fruits offer optimal health benefits. Additionally, they can be enjoyed in various other forms, such as smoothies, freshly squeezed juices, and delectable fruit salads. Instead of eating unhealthy and processed snacks that give you nothing, fruits are the best choice to make them part of your daily food intake.

Legumes:

Legumes are as healthy as vegetables. You can cook them anytime you want. They have a longer shelf life than other grains. They include lentils, peas, and beans. Legumes are widely consumed worldwide, and their many health benefits are widely acknowledged. They are the nutritional powerhouse. Eating them on a regular basis is a great way to lose and maintain a healthy weight. High in protein, legumes serve as an excellent meat substitute and are favored by vegetarians worldwide, along with vegetables, beans, fruits, and nuts.

Legumes are not only tasty; they are also easily available and easy to cook, making them an ideal choice together with vegetables. Together with proteins, they are rich in fiber. They are low in fat and, at the same time, packed with essential vitamins, antioxidants, and minerals. Legumes have probiotic fiber, which is good for gut health. Eating legumes is also good for healthy gut bacteria.

Their contribution to weight loss is undeniable. They are a great source of energy and nutrition, which proves their healthy qualities. They contribute to an extended sensation of satiety. Also, they help maintain healthy blood sugar levels. Their high protein content aids in boosting metabolism. There are different ways to cook them, depending on individual taste. Some of the healthy options include soups, salads, stews, curries, salads, and stir-fries. Therefore, making legumes part of your diet ensures good health and high energy levels. **Beans:**

Though beans and legumes are related, they are not exactly the same. Beans typically have a larger size in comparison to lentils. Beans, much like vegetables and lentils, are popularly consumed for their health benefits and delicious taste. The commonly consumed beans are pinto beans, kidney beans, black beans, lima beans, and chickpeas. There are many varieties found in these beans. All of them are equally healthy, tasty, and high in proteins.

Beans are prepared in various ways, similar to lentils. They can be cooked into stews, incorporated into salads, or used in curries. While they are often consumed in canned packaging for convenience, the healthier choice is to cook them in their natural form to retain their nutritious properties. They are high in fiber, magnesium, vitamin B, and protein. Making them part of your daily meals makes them a healthy and tasty option to help you lose weight quickly.

Low-Fat Dairy Products:

Low-fat dairy products are a vital part of your daily food intake. Dairy products, vital for maintaining good health, are included in this diet due to their nutritional value. They help with feelings of fullness and have a calming effect. They are very helpful in losing and maintaining a healthy weight. They are a much better option compared to full-fat dairy products like full-cream milk and butter. Healthier choices include 1%-fat low-fat milk, low-fat yogurt, and skim milk-based low-fat cheeses like cheddar, mozzarella, and cottage cheese.

These dairy products are low in calories yet rich in nutritional value, offering significant health benefits. They are abundant in proteins, calcium, vitamin D, probiotics, and minerals. These properties are good for the health of bones, teeth, eyes, and brains. Low-fat dairy products boost metabolism and aid in appetite regulation. Probiotics that are in yogurt are beneficial for gut health. Regular consumption of dairy products ensures good health and plays a part in weight loss.

Eggs:

Eggs do have an impact on weight loss. They have a high protein content, which helps with metabolism and weight management.

The low calorie count makes it a safer choice when it comes to weight loss. At the same time, they are a nutrient-dense food, which makes them a good source of essential vitamins and minerals like vitamin B, D, and iron. Various types of eggs are available for consumption, including duck, goose, guinea fowl, chicken, and ostrich eggs. Indeed, chicken eggs are the most commonly consumed and popular choice among consumers. They are available throughout the year. Healthy options include eggs from free-range or domestic hens, known for their filling properties. You eat a couple of eggs, feel full, and immediately notice energy in your body.

The best time to eat eggs is at breakfast. The body needs a lot of energy during the early hours of the day. Therefore, to give your body enough energy for the whole day, there is nothing better than a couple of eggs. The great thing about eggs is that you can prepare them in different ways, like fried eggs, poached eggs, boiled eggs, or different types of omelets. While you are losing weight, never eat them in the evening, as that can cause weight gain.

Making them part of your daily breakfast is a wise decision. Choose eggs that are rich in omega-3 fatty acids to get the maximum health benefits. Combining eggs with low-fat dairy products, healthy grains like buckwheat, dry or fresh fruits, pure juices, and nuts makes your breakfast super healthy, fills you, provides you lots of energy for the whole day, and gives you a great start with a good mood.

Lean Meat:

When it comes to meat, there is nothing better than lean meat for weight-loss purposes. White meat is known for its low fat content and health properties. This allows you to still enjoy meat, but the key is to choose healthy options that support your overall health and weight-loss goals. The good thing about lean meat is that it is easy and quick to prepare, and there are many ways to cook it, notably in the oven, stews, curries, grilled, BBQ, and with rice and vegetables.

When it comes to lean meat, the ideal choice is chicken or turkey breast, as both are low in fat and calories. They are filling and tasty. Avoid consuming fried chicken, including the chicken skin.

Then there are some varieties of fish to choose from. The best ones are salmon, cod, tuna, tilapia, and carp. Fish can also be prepared in a variety of ways, and it is a delicious option. Its high protein content makes it an ideal choice among the low-calorie options mentioned above.

Fatty and processed meats are detrimental to health and a significant contributor to weight gain. The rich nutrients, minerals, vitamin B12, zinc, and iron make them an ideal part of this weight-loss diet. The best choice is lean meat sourced from free-range and grass-fed poultry, which boasts superior health benefits compared to commercially produced meat.

Dry Fruits:

Dry fruits are no less beneficial for health than fresh fruits. Just because they are dry does not mean that they are not healthy. They are nutritious and an excellent healthy snack option, beneficial for weight loss. There is a wide variety of dry fruits available, like dry figs, bananas, mangos, apricots, dates, plums, raisins, and many more. Everyone likes to try some dry fruits due to their good taste.

Dry fruits are full of antioxidants that help reduce inflammation. They are high in fiber and make the digestion process easy. They are naturally sweet and can be eaten as a dessert after the meal to help the digestion process, making them a much better choice than those desserts that are made from refined sugar. Most of these dry fruits are low in calories. Though dates are high in sweetness and therefore should be eaten in moderation,.

Seeds:

Seeds are a healthy food packed with nutrients, fiber, proteins, and healthy fats. Additionally, they boast abundant antioxidants while being low in calories. Making them part of your diet helps reduce weight. They help strengthen the metabolism. The healthy fats found in these seeds are generally beneficial for health. They are also good for the heart. Most of these seeds are low in calories, which makes them a healthy and guilt-free snack.

Many seeds are used to extract oil, and some of these oils, like sunflower oil, are commonly used for cooking. Other oils that are famous for their health properties are black seed oil, mustard oil, pumpkin seed oil, sesame oil, and flaxseed oil. These seeds should be used in moderation and according to your dietary needs. They are tasty, healthy, and good for weight loss.

Nuts:

Nuts are highly tasty and, at the same time, healthy. Nuts are a popular food, and there are many varieties, each with a different and unique taste, all of which are healthy to consume. These nuts include Brazil nuts, pecans, almonds, walnuts, hazelnuts, cashews, pine nuts, and pistachios. Though peanuts are technically legumes, they are consumed as nuts and are quite popular among people due to their taste and affordability.

Nuts are used in cooking, oil extraction for various purposes, baking, and are widely consumed as snacks. In some countries, their consumption increases during the winter months. They are rich in healthy fats and can help keep you full and satisfied. They are so tasty that when you start eating them, it's hard to stop. Nut trees are found in various parts of the world. Nuts are exported in large quantities to different countries.

They are a good source of protein. Rich in fiber and antioxidants while low in carbohydrates, nuts are healthy foods. Rich in fiber and antioxidants while low in carbohydrates, nuts are healthy foods. However, consume them in moderation. Their nutritional properties make them beneficial.

Grains:

Grains are widely consumed worldwide. On top of the list are wheat, rice, and corn. Grains are a staple food in many cuisines and are harvested each year in large quantities. Some grains are very helpful in losing and maintaining a healthy weight. They are high in fiber, rich in nutrients, low in calories, and satisfying. Grains are used in bread making, creating various snacks, bakery products, desserts, and sweets. Rice is a staple ingredient in numerous dishes. It's hard to imagine life without grains for many people, as they are an essential part of their daily food consumption.

They are packed with vitamins, fiber, and nutrients. They offer a low-calorie option while providing antioxidants. That makes them a healthy food for dieting. There are numerous ways to prepare various foods with these grains. Some of the grains are light yet filling, which makes you feel fuller for a long time and reduces the likelihood of overeating. The good thing about these grains is that they are a great combination with different healthy foods, like vegetables, legumes, and beans. That makes them a healthy food and an ideal choice for losing weight.

Chapter 5: Diet Plan

The diet plan consists of three meals a day. Breakfast, lunch, and dinner. The main meals of the day consist of breakfast and lunch, while dinner should consist of a minimum amount of food, which should consist of light foods like salad or fruits. Once you've familiarized yourself with the approved foods in this diet, grasping its concept becomes straightforward. The diet is primarily based on light meals complemented by salads and fruits, accompanied by water or fruit juices. This combination serves as an efficient source of nourishment and energy while minimizing the intake of excess calories, facilitating rapid weight loss.

What makes this diet highly effective is the emphasis on what to eat, when to eat, and how to eat food to get the best results. Timing plays a crucial role in this diet, as the meal schedule is divided into three parts of the day. Breakfast, lunch, and dinner. The major food portions should be breakfast and lunch to provide the body with energy when it needs it the most, and that is during the day when you are physically active, either at work or some other activity. The dinner must be very light and minimal; avoid eating food in the late evening hours to give the body and digestive system the rest they need.

Consuming food outside of designated mealtimes is prohibited to prevent overeating and provide your digestive system with adequate rest. Eating between meals is one of the main factors that contribute to weight gain. Therefore, consistently snacking throughout the day, especially when not hungry, can significantly contribute to weight gain. Eating only during your meal times sufficiently provides you with enough energy and nourishment that you don't feel the need to eat anything until your next meal time.

By consuming a substantial amount of food during breakfast, you should feel satiated until lunchtime. Similarly, at lunch, eating enough food to sustain you until dinner ensures that you maintain energy levels throughout the day. Adjust meal portions according to your appetite. When you follow this diet pattern, reducing weight quickly becomes a reality. Eat according to your appetite, ensuring you consume enough to satisfy your hunger and sustain your energy levels, particularly during the day.

The evening is not a good time for eating food due to the risk of gaining weight; therefore, this diet recommends only light meals before 7 p.m. That is because when we are physically active during the day, we burn calories quickly and efficiently, while in the evening hours we slow down, and the process of burning calories also slows down, thus making it easier to gain weight from the consumption of foods during the evening hours.

Since it's a gluten-free diet, you must avoid any food made from wheat, such as bread. Instead, you combine your meals with rice or other grains, like buckwheat. The meals in this diet are designed with moderation and a balanced combination of healthy foods in mind. This combination works effectively to help rapidly reduce your weight.

The breakfast should be about the same portion as your lunch. The logic behind this is that the body requires energy in the early hours of the day. During the morning hours, as you prepare for work, commute to your workplace, and engage in early work tasks, Thus, a good portion of breakfast provides you with enough nourishment and energy that you don't feel hungry until lunch time. This way, a good breakfast provides your body with comfort and saves you from feeling uneasy due to the urge to eat something, thus making your day stress-free and energetic.

For a solid, healthy breakfast to kickstart your day, include low-dairy products, eggs, fruits, pure fruit juices, and nuts. A nourishing breakfast sets the tone for your entire day, both mentally and physically. It's crucial to begin your day well, as it sets the tone for the rest of the day. With adequate rest for your body and digestive system overnight, you wake up refreshed and with a healthy appetite for breakfast. Eating a satisfying breakfast will leave you feeling calm and energetic throughout the morning, enabling you to tackle your work with a positive attitude. That is what a good and healthy breakfast does for you. This sets the stage for a pleasant, energetic, and stress-free day overall.

By the time lunch time comes, it's time to have a good-sized portion of lunch that should include a good combination of foods from this diet's list to provide you with the energy and nourishment your body needs until dinner time. For instance, when you have a meal with rice, the rice portion should not exceed one-third of your plate. Ideally, one part of the plate should be rice, another part should include vegetables, legumes, or beans, and the remaining part should consist of salad. This balanced meal can also include soup, fruits, water, or pure fruit juice. Good-quality boiled rice is a healthy food that is fat-free and easily digestible. The preferred choice is brown rice, but since rice consumption in this diet is moderate, you have the flexibility to choose any type of rice without concern.

For lunch, you have the freedom to choose from the permitted list of foods. For instance, you can choose from options like chicken, turkey breast, or fish, which can be accompanied by rice. Legumes or beans with rice—these combinations of different foods will make your meals tasty and enjoyable. Make salads, soups, and fruits an essential part of your meals, as they are very light and easily digestible. The light meals are the ones that are the game changers; in other words, they are miracle foods. These light meals are fat-free, low in calories, easy to digest, and filling, thus making them extremely healthy and helpful for rapid weight loss.

The dinner must be minimal, which means you should only eat something light like salad, fruits, or some nuts to satisfy yourself and prepare for the evening rest. The earlier in the evening you eat your dinner with the minimum amount of food, the better for you. Your digestive system requires ample time to rest overnight to prepare for a substantial breakfast in the morning. Consuming a light dinner around 6 to 7 p.m. is considered the healthiest approach to eating your evening meal. Avoid eating anything after this time. The more hours you get a break between your dinner time and your next morning breakfast, the more quickly you lose weight. This is what really makes the difference. The type of food, the amount of food, the timing of your meals, and the break between meals are the main factors that, when you adjust to them, will get you the best results for losing weight and maintaining it thereafter. Make soups and salads an essential part of your daily meals. Indeed, they complement your meal wonderfully while contributing to its healthiness. Soups are healthy, easy to digest, and tasty. Soups are low-calorie yet filling and prepared relatively quickly compared to other foods, making them an excellent source of nourishment. They typically consist of vegetables and legume-based liquids rich in fiber, providing the body with essential energy.

Food that consists of liquids is much healthier, lighter, and easily digestible. Consuming soups prepared in a healthy manner can work wonders for the body, including aiding in weight reduction. Soups should be prepared with moderation in salt, spices, and cooking oil to ensure a balance between taste and health. The primary focus should always be on the nutritional value of the food rather than solely on taste. Overemphasizing taste can lead to the consumption of foods that are high in flavor but detrimental to health. It's crucial to avoid the mistake of indulging in processed foods that prioritize taste over nutritional value, as they pose a threat to your well-being.

Chapter 6: Bad Habits and Unhealthy Practices

Bad habits and unhealthy practices are responsible for weight gain. Any bad habit has negative consequences. Unhealthy habits not only impact health but also incur financial costs. They waste time and energy and give you nothing in return. People develop bad habits over time and start doing things that create problems for them. These problems are usually not short-term problems, and getting rid of them is nothing less than a headache.

Usually, people find it hard to change their bad habits, and this struggle may take years. Therefore, it is important at first not to adopt bad habits, and for the ones you already have, the only solution is to overcome them for your own benefit. Smoking, substance abuse, late sleep, and overworking all contribute to an unhealthy lifestyle. Living a clean life free from bad habits and addictions is a great quality that makes a real difference in our lives. Below is a list of some bad habits and unhealthy practices:

Overeating:

Overeating is a recipe for disaster. The body has its capacity, and when you misuse it, you pay the price for that. Eating more than your body needs is indeed overeating. Processing foods consumed in large quantities gives your digestive system a hard time. Your body is not able to cope with an influx of calories. Overeating affects vital organs such as the heart, kidneys, and liver.

Initially, the body exerts its strength to combat the effects, but over time, it may succumb, leading to various health issues. Continuing to eat food when you have already eaten your normal portion of a meal is what creates obesity. It's like forcing yourself to do something that is unnatural and unhealthy.

Putting an excessive amount of food on your plate and feeling compelled to finish it, even when you're already full and craving more, indicates overeating. Ignoring signals to stop eating after consuming a normal portion can lead to various health issues. The only way to stop overeating is to have self-control and immediately stop eating once your appetite is over. You can do so by getting yourself busy with some work so that you have no time to think about eating more without an appetite.

Mindless Eating:

Eating food without an appetite is a mindless act. It's like chain smoking; you finish smoking one cigarette, and soon you start smoking another one. However, people keep eating something all the time; it's like a never-ending process that continues the whole day, right until the time you go to bed. Whether it's potato chips, candies, chocolate, peanuts, or whatever appeals to you, you keep eating them while you are sitting in front of a computer, TV, reading a book, or just doing anything else.

Snacking often becomes a way to add enjoyment to activities. Once the habit of snacking while engaged in activities becomes established, breaking it can prove challenging. This way, you keep adding calories to your body, while these excessive calories are adding fat to your body. There is no machine that can tell you how many calories are piling up in your body when you are snacking, so it's you who have to understand that whatever you eat will produce some calories, and the more you eat, the more calories are piling up in your body.

To eliminate mindless eating, avoid all snacks. Don't keep any snacks in your home or take them to work. When you don't have snacks at home, you'll only eat during mealtime. By getting accustomed to eating only during meals, mindless eating will no longer be a concern.

Skipping Meals:

Skipping meals is a huge mistake; it disturbs the whole body's internal system. The body relies on the digestion process to obtain energy and nutrients to function. Skipping meals disrupts the body's internal system and the digestive routine it's accustomed to.

Skipping meals can lead to feelings of discomfort and stress due to hunger. So whatever you do while you are hungry makes you nervous, stressed, and uncomfortable. You require peace while working, but when you're not feeling normal and unable to perform tasks properly, it diminishes the quality of your work and reduces your concentration on the task at hand.

Skipping meals leads to overeating because when you eat food when you are too hungry, not only do you eat quickly, you don't chew food properly, and it's nothing more than a stressful experience that is bad for your health. Usually people skip their breakfast when they wake up late or, for some reason, don't have time to eat it. They go to work and feel stressed and uncomfortable due to a lack of energy and hunger. This not only disturbs your work routine but also affects you negatively throughout the day.

Eating meals on time means managing a healthy eating regime that benefits your digestive system and body as a whole. That is how you prevent overeating. Consuming healthy and balanced meals regularly helps prevent weight gain and maintain stable hunger and energy levels.

Improper Eating:

There is another problem with gaining weight: not eating what you have to eat. So when there is a time for breakfast, you have to eat

a proper breakfast that can provide you with a good start to the

day and fulfill your energy needs leading up to lunch time.

Therefore, consuming only a cup of tea or coffee, or eating too

little, can result in feelings of stress and hunger, often leading to

overeating during lunch.

Similarly, if you only eat breakfast and neglect to have a proper

lunch or skip it altogether, you may overeat during dinner. This can

result in weight gain, stomach discomfort, and even reflux during

sleep. Properly eating meals during breakfast, lunch, and dinner

times helps prevent such issues, ensuring you eat appropriately.

Moreover, avoid consuming food that doesn't match your appetite.

For example, opting for a snack instead of a regular portion during

lunch won't provide your body with the necessary nutrients,

potentially leading to overeating later on. Therefore, eat according

to your appetite and meal times. Proper eating means taking care

of your health and living a stress-free life.

Chapter 7: Herbs and Spices for Weight Loss

There are some herbs and spices that are helpful for weight loss. Due to their health properties, their role in weight loss cannot be ignored. Their addition to the diet makes the weight-loss journey easier. Nature has given us so many precious gifts, and if we use them wisely, we can benefit from them all our lives. There is no shortage of means and possibilities to improve our lives; therefore, we should be grateful for all of nature's gifts.

The spices and herbs are as beneficial as other natural things. Below are some of the herbs and spices that can be used for weight loss purposes:

Ginger:

Ginger is a spice that is cultivated in warm climates. It has a unique smell and taste. It is widely used in cooking. It helps enhance the aroma and flavor of various dishes. Ginger is good at burning fat and removing toxins from the body. Drinking boiled ginger water has a relaxing effect, and its use in winter warms up our bodies. Eating ginger regulates appetite and helps the digestion process. It has been used for many centuries as medicine and in various remedies. It is easily available throughout the year. Drinking a glass of boiled ginger water every day helps reduce weight. Therefore, its daily use is recommended in moderation.

Garlic:

Just like ginger, garlic is widely used in cooking. Garlic is rich in many healthy properties. Garlic is antiviral, anti-bacterial, and antifungal. Garlic strengthens metabolism, suppresses appetite, and helps burn body fat. It's very helpful in regulating insulin levels in the body. It has healing properties for the body. It can help lower cholesterol levels, making it a great food for heart health. Regular use of garlic strengthens immunity and helps fight against seasonal illnesses like flu and coughing. Garlic also has anti-inflammatory properties, which could help alleviate conditions like arthritis and asthma. Considering its many health benefits, garlic is indeed a great herb overall for health.

Fenugreek:

Fenugreek belongs to the legume family. Fenugreek seeds are used in cooking to enhance the flavor of food. Fenugreek is helpful in controlling appetite, thus preventing overeating. Fenugreek seeds are good for digestion, especially treating constipation, bloating, and diarrhea. Its use is also helpful in diabetes for lowering blood sugar levels. Fenugreek also has anti-inflammatory properties, which may help with arthritis. It also contributes to the health and vitality of hair and skin. Due to its unique features, the use of fenugreek is indeed beneficial for maintaining good health.

Turmeric:

Turmeric is a wonderful spice that has many uses. Turmeric has incredible healing properties. Not only is it a widely used spice in cooking, but it also plays a role in preventing many diseases. Its yellow color makes it easily recognizable. In many cuisines, the use of turmeric is a must, especially in curries. It brings color, taste, and smell to stews and curries. Curcumin, found in turmeric, is anti-inflammatory and very helpful in arthritis. Turmeric burns fat and is helpful for weight loss. It strengthens immunity and is good for the skin. It is frequently incorporated into home remedies due to its beneficial properties.

Black Pepper:

Black pepper is a well-known spice that is widely used in cooking. It enhances the flavor of food. The powerful compound called piperine not only enhances flavor but also aids in burning fat in the body. It is considered more healthy than red chili peppers due to its health properties. It has numerous health benefits. It contains antioxidants that help prevent cell damage. It reduces bloating and gas in the stomach and helps absorb nutrients. Black pepper is also helpful in reducing inflammation and arthritis. It helps prevent the growth of bacteria. Black pepper is also beneficial for weight loss.

Cayenne Pepper:

Cayenne pepper belongs to the chili pepper family. It is extensively used in culinary preparations as a spice. It brings flavor and color to dishes. The capsaicin compound in cayenne pepper has many health benefits. It is a strong fat burner, and its regular use helps lower weight. It's useful for strengthening the metabolism. It can also help contain hunger. It is helpful to digest food. It is used in various remedies for different health conditions; its moderate use is beneficial for health.

Oregano:

Oregano is a flavorful herb that can help with weight loss. It's easy to find and use in cooking, and it adds a delicious taste to many dishes. But beyond its great flavor, oregano has some surprising benefits for weight loss. It's packed with antioxidants, which are compounds that help combat inflammation in the body. When your body is less inflamed, it can function better and may even burn calories more efficiently. Oregano is also a natural diuretic, meaning it helps your body get rid of excess water weight. Plus, it's low in calories itself, so you can use it to flavor your food without adding many extra calories. Oregano possesses antimicrobial properties, meaning it can help maintain the health of your digestive system. When your gut is happy and working well, it's easier to maintain a healthy weight. Don't forget to sprinkle some oregano while cooking—it might just help you shed some extra pounds.

Fennel:

Fennel is a versatile and flavorful herb with numerous health benefits. It has a distinct licorice-like taste and can be used in various culinary dishes, both savory and sweet. Beyond its culinary uses, fennel offers several health benefits, including aiding in digestion. It contains compounds that can help reduce bloating, gas, and indigestion, making it a popular choice for after-dinner teas or snacks. Additionally, fennel is rich in antioxidants and fiber, which can support overall digestive health and promote regular bowel movements, potentially aiding in weight-loss efforts. Some studies suggest that fennel may also have antimicrobial properties, helping to combat harmful bacteria in the gut. Overall, incorporating fennel into your diet can be a flavorful way to support digestive health and potentially contribute to weight management.

Cinnamon:

Cinnamon is renowned for its warm and sweet flavor, making it a beloved addition to both cooking and baking. Beyond its delicious taste, cinnamon offers numerous health benefits, including potential support for weight loss. One of its key benefits is its ability to help regulate blood sugar levels. Cinnamon contains compounds that can improve insulin sensitivity, which may help control blood sugar spikes after meals and reduce cravings for sugary foods. By stabilizing blood sugar levels, cinnamon may also help prevent energy crashes and reduce overall calorie intake. Additionally, cinnamon has been shown to have anti-inflammatory properties, which can support overall health and potentially aid in weight loss by reducing inflammation in the body. Incorporating cinnamon into your diet, whether sprinkled on oatmeal, added to coffee, or used in cooking, can be a tasty way to enjoy its potential weight management benefits.

Cumin:

Cumin is a versatile spice that not only adds a distinctive flavor to dishes but also offers several potential health benefits, including support for weight loss. This spice is commonly used in cuisines around the world and has a warm, earthy taste with a slightly nutty undertone. One of the ways cumin may aid in weight loss is by boosting metabolism. Some studies suggest that cumin can increase the rate at which the body burns calories, potentially leading to enhanced fat loss over time. Additionally, cumin may help reduce appetite and food intake. It contains compounds that have been shown to suppress appetite and promote feelings of fullness, which can help prevent overeating and support weight management efforts. Furthermore, cumin has been linked to improved digestion and reduced bloating, which can contribute to a flatter stomach and overall weight loss success. Incorporating cumin into your diet, whether by sprinkling it on roasted vegetables, adding it to soups and stews, or using it to season meats, can be a flavorful way to enjoy its potential weight-loss benefits.

Cardamom:

Cardamom is a fragrant spice that offers not only a unique flavor but also potential health benefits, including support for weight loss. This spice has a sweet, spicy taste with floral undertones and is commonly used in both sweet and savory dishes. One way cardamom may aid in weight loss is by boosting metabolism. Some research suggests that compounds found in cardamom can help increase the body's metabolic rate, leading to more efficient calorie burning and potential fat loss. Additionally, cardamom has been shown to have diuretic properties, meaning it can help rid the body of excess water weight, which may result in temporary weight loss. Furthermore, cardamom may help improve digestion and reduce bloating, which can contribute to a flatter stomach and a feeling of lightness. Incorporating cardamom into your diet, whether by adding it to baked goods, sprinkling it over oatmeal, or using it in savory dishes like curries and rice pilafs, can be a delicious way to enjoy its potential weight-management benefits.

Chapter 8: Healthy Tips

All the little steps we take to take care of our health all add up to benefit us tremendously. As long as we don't stop neglecting our health, we cannot expect to be totally healthy and happy. Happiness and good health are both related to each other, because when one or both of these things are missing from our lives, we cannot live a normal and meaningful life.

Here are some helpful tips that are not only good for your health but also helpful in reducing and maintaining a healthy weight:

Drink Plenty of Liquids:

Fruit and vegetable juices, preferably freshly made with water, are a great source of vitamins. They do three main things brilliantly: they keep you dehydrated, provide you with a healthy supply of vitamins and nutrition, and detox your body. Thanks to fruit juices, you can avoid consuming unhealthy drinks loaded with refined sugar, which can contribute to weight gain without providing your body with the essential nutrition it needs. Those who drink plenty of water and pure juice are healthy, have stronger stamina, and have a high energy level all the time.

Drinking enough fluids helps control body temperature, carry nutrients, and flush out waste. Furthermore, drinking enough water can aid in weight management, improve skin health, and support kidney function. In addition to fruit and vegetable juices, other low-calorie drinks like water, herbal tea, and low-fat milk can contribute to a healthy hydration routine. Stay away from sugary drinks and caffeine, which can have negative effects when consumed regularly. By making water and nutrient-rich beverages part of your daily drinking regime, you'll be well on your way to maintaining adequate hydration and reaping the benefits.

Good Sleep:

Sleep is a time when we are able to get rest and recharge our bodies. Without a regular, good amount of sleep, it is not possible to carry on daily tasks and other activities normally. Poor-quality sleep is often the culprit behind low energy levels, fatigue, and weakened immunity. Individuals who consistently get insufficient sleep may age more quickly and develop wrinkles on their faces prematurely compared to their peers.

The best way to make the most of the day is to go to sleep early. When you go to sleep early, you use the time that nature has set for us to rest. Daytime is for work, and nighttime is for sleep. So when you go to sleep early, you get up early. When you get up early, you have enough time to do things in peace without hurrying or worrying.

When you start early, it enables you to do many things and still find some free time because you are able to finish your daily assignments earlier. This also allows you to make time for exercise and other physical activities; therefore, going to bed early yields numerous positive outcomes overall.

Reduce Stress:

Stress is so common these days that even finding a few moments of peace and calmness seems hard. The hectic life, together with the excessive use of technology and lack of a natural environment, is making life stressful. In order to reduce stress, it is important to get rid of those things that are the source of stress. These include excessive use of phones and the internet, stressful work, and a lack of physical activity.

Reduce the use of the phone. Avoid constantly checking your phone every few minutes to see if you've received a call, email, or text message. Just ignore it as much as you can. Phones have become a significant source of stress in modern times, with many people mindlessly and excessively using them throughout the day. They start their day with a phone, and the last thing they do before going to sleep is to finally take another look at their phone.

Another significant source of stress is the excessive use of the internet. Whether you use it on your smart phone or on other devices, you are unnecessarily consuming information that you really don't need. People have made these things part of their lives unnecessarily by cutting ties with each other in real life. Instead of spending time with each other or taking part in some healthy and interesting activities, they are wasting our lives each day on the internet and getting nothing out of it. Stress can only be reduced by addressing its root causes and taking action against the factors in your life that contribute to it.

Get Rid of Clutter:

Clutter is quite a common problem these days due to excessive consumerism and the influence of media and advertisements. There are many problems related to clutter, like stress, time waste, obesity, shopping addiction, and depression. Clutter is not limited to physical items. There are other forms of clutter, like too many thoughts, activities, worries, and so on, and all of them have a negative influence on our lives.

To bring normality to life, it is important to get rid of all forms of clutter so you can pay attention to the issues that are important to you. The time you save can be channeled towards enhancing your life and attending to essential tasks. With more time, energy, and peace at your disposal, you'll be better equipped to leverage them for your own benefit. Losing weight is one of the things you can easily achieve by getting rid of clutter. Eating healthy and using your free time to exercise will immediately start to help you reduce weight. Those who get rid of clutter have much better lives and health compared to those who live with it.

Decluttering has a strong impact on both physical and mental well-being. By removing clutter, you create space for new experiences, relationships, and personal growth. You can start by decluttering small areas, like your desk or a single shelf, and work your way up to other parts of your house. Don't forget to declutter digital spaces, like your phone and computer, to reduce distractions and increase productivity.

Clutter extends beyond the physical realm and can have detrimental effects on emotional and mental well-being, potentially leading to behaviors like overeating or consuming unhealthy foods, which can contribute to weight gain. So don't let negative thoughts, worries, and emotions weigh you down. Practice mindfulness, meditation, and self-reflection to clear your mind and heart. By releasing clutter in all its forms, you'll create a more peaceful, organized, and healthy life for your own benefit.

Connect with nature:

If there is something that can help us a lot these days, it is spending time in nature. The hectic and stressful life is tiring us, draining all of our energies, and depriving us of happiness and peace that we badly need. There is stress and worry every day, and finding a balance is getting harder and harder. To initiate positive changes in your life, consider spending time in nature to allow your mind and body to relax and rejuvenate.

The greenery, the calmness, and the freshness all have a healing effect on the mind and the body. Nature offers significant relief to a weary body burdened by stress, noise, and the frantic pace of modern life, which profoundly affects people's well-being. When you experience tranquility in nature, your mind operates more effectively, your body gains energy, and, as a result, you become more physically active, aiding in calorie burn and weight reduction.

Spending time in nature has clear and sound benefits, including reduced inflammation, improved mood, and increased vitamin D levels. Being in nature also disconnects you from the constant dependency on technology and reconnects you with your inner self. Spend more time in parks, hike in the woods, or simply sit outside and get some sunshine.

Allow nature to positively impact your life and alleviate your tensions. You'll experience a sense of renewal and rejuvenation that will make you feel totally different. Indeed, nature is a powerful tool for improving physical and mental health. Make it a priority to spend time outdoors, and you'll start to notice the positive effects on your body and mind. Observe and enjoy the beauty and tranquility of nature, and let it make you a happy person.

Eat in peace:

The fast-paced nature of modern life has made even the simple act of eating peacefully a challenge for many people, as they find themselves constantly rushing through tasks. You must eat in a quiet and peaceful environment so that there is no stress or distraction that can affect your meal time. Minimize distractions during meals by switching off your phone and avoiding activities like talking on the phone, reading, or watching screens. These habits can negatively impact your digestive system and overall health.

Eat your food in small portions and chew it slowly and thoroughly. When you eat fast, you don't chew it thoroughly, and you end up eating more than you should. Eating fast is not a natural or civilized way of eating. When you eat slowly, you eat only the amount of food that your body needs, thus preventing overeating. It all makes the digestive process quick and healthy.

The plates should be white or light colors; it has a calming effect. Don't eat in darkness. Eat food in a relaxed mood. Don't think about anything; eat quietly, and keep looking at your food in your mind so you don't think about anything else than food. Drinking a bit of water or some juice before the meal relaxes the stomach and prepares it for the digestion process. Adding a sweet touch to the end of a meal with fresh or dried fruit is a great way to satisfy cravings while still maintaining a healthy diet. It is helpful in the digestion process.

After the meal, try to get a few minutes of rest instead of immediately engaging in something; all of these measures are helpful for your digestion and health. Do not take a bath immediately after the meal. Don't lay down on the bed or engage in some sports. Let the digestion process happen in peace, so your body benefits accordingly.

Live Healthy:

Life is a precious gift, and we must take care of it as much as we can. Whatever you do, do it in a way that contributes to your good health. Whether it is food, working, sleeping, hobbies, or lifestyle, do them all in a healthy manner so they all make you healthy and strong. Focusing solely on one aspect of life while neglecting others is a common mistake that often yields unfavorable results. Overworking without allocating time for family and relaxation can lead to health problems and overall dissatisfaction.

So the appropriate way is to make healthy choices about everything you do. Your health must be your priority, because if you are not healthy, you will not be able to manage your life in a normal way. It is not possible to enjoy life with poor health. In order to bring balance to life, one must do things moderately and in a healthy manner. Give time to everything: your family, friends, fitness, exercising, relaxation, travel, hobbies, and so on. This way, you will have a much more balanced, healthy, and happy life.

By adopting a smart approach to health, you'll experience numerous benefits that extend beyond physical well-being. Your mental and emotional health will also flourish, leading to enhanced resilience, happier relationships, and a greater sense of purpose for life. Small changes can add up over time, so start with manageable steps towards a healthier lifestyle.

Enjoy your journey towards wellness, and make the most of every day of your life along the way. With each healthy choice, you're investing in your long-term happiness and vitality. The thing to remember is that it's just a continuous process, and it's okay to take things one step at a time instead of multitasking. By prioritizing your health and well-being, you'll unlock a more fulfilling life that creates positivity and energy.

Enjoy Life:

Life is short. It's not just about working, making money, and buying stuff. People forget important things and end up making bad choices, keeping their minds narrow. Having a good time in life doesn't always require a lot of money. It shouldn't be the main focus or the top priority. There are other things that are more important than money, like health, family, friends, happiness, and peace. Doing things with happiness, joy, and fun makes life interesting and enjoyable. Whatever you do, do it happily. Don't miss an opportunity to smile and bring a smile to the faces of others.

Share whatever you have with others. Take care of yourself and others. Be part of the community. Have a positive attitude. Look around and learn from others. Participate in good causes. Spend time with people you like. So the bottom line is not to miss any opportunity to enjoy life and find happiness, because that is what life is all about.

The End.

www.ingramcontent.com/pod-product-compliance
Lightning Source LLC
Chambersburg PA
CBHW050817250726
48653CB00006B/2280